Alkaline Diet

Discover How To Alkalize Your Body With This PH Balance Diet And Super foods Guide To Boost Your Energy.

(How To Alkalize To Lose Weight And Boost Your Vitality)

Emanuel Meadows

TABLE OF CONTENT

Introduction

The alkaline diet is noticeably distinct from all of those fad diets and eating fads that mislead people into a false sense of health. It is not based on pseudoscience or current food fads, but rather on empirical evidence and common sense. Each and every individual who strives to achieve their body's optimal pH balance can reap astounding benefits. You could fill one of those positions. You should revitalise your health, restore your vitality, look absolutely incredible, and rid yourself of those difficult-to-change health conditions. You know the ones I'm talking about: the skin conditions that do not respond to treatment, the IBS symptoms that constantly flare up, the allergies, fatigue, and sluggish thought processes.

Various studies have found that rats fed an alkalizing rlant-based diet lost weight, lowered their blood pressure, and were cured of a variety of health issues, in addition to turning off a number of genes involved in the development of cancer. We simply cannot disregard the incredible long-term benefits that this way of life provides.

An alkaline diet encourages the consumption of fruits, vegetables, nuts, and legumes while discouraging the consumption of acidic foods; these eating patterns have been repeatedly linked to health benefits. But there is no evidence that you benefit from these foods because they alter the pH level of the body.

Your bodu's pH level is astuallu veru finelu tuned. Your digestive organs are more acidic, which aids in the digestion of proteins passing through them.

Pancreatic fluid and bile in the gut tend to be more acidic, neutralising acidic and acidic digestion. Vaginal fluid typically contains rrettu asds, which inhibit the growth of harmful bastera. The rH level of urine fluctuates between acidic and basic, depending on what must be flushed out of the body in order to neutralise it.

What is Alkalinity?

Alkalinity indicates that a substance has a pH greater than 7. The human body is slightly alkaline by nature, with a blood pH of approximately 7.8 . The acidity of the tomash enables it to digest food. The pH of saliva and urine varies based on diet, metabolic rate, and other factors.
Explanation pertaining to this book:
Liquids can be measured according to their alkalinity and acidity using a scale known as the rH value, which ranges

from 0 to 2 8 . 0 to 7 indicates acidity, and anything above 7 indicates alkalinity.

Every living thing must have optimal rH balance in order to live healthily and perform optimally. Fish require water with the lowest pH levels to survive, whereas algae will flourish in pH-balanced water. Of course, the exact wording is arrle to our bodies as well. To function optimally, our blood, urine, and fluids require a rH value of approximately 7.6 610 , which is slightly on the alkaline side of the scale. When the body's acidity-alkalinity balance is optimal, it is less susceptible to lowered immunity, chronic disease, and cellular damage.

Our bodies have evolved to constantly shift and adjust to maintain homeostasis (balance) in all body parts, and our rH levels are no exception. Under natural conditions, it performs exceptionally well.

Not everyone is confronted with this issue under 'natural sondton'; it may have occurred as a result of the following.

Processed foods: the high-sugar, high-saturated-fat, refined-sugar meals that make us gradually sicker and sicker. And we ubjest our bode to a load of toxic environmental factors: unnatural levels of tre, abusing ourelve with tmulant, alcohol, and drug, surrounding ourselves with retsde, rolluton, and chemicals, and depriving ourselves of sleep; yet we wonder why we don't feel or look our best.

Unfavorable conduct: We increase the acidity level in our systems, overloading the detoxfson and alkalizing abilities of the body and creating a burden of inflammation and oxidative stress - ush an asne, kn deae, bowel problems, tumour, mgrane, leerng trouble, bran fog, exse weght, infertility, and eventually something more serious like heart disease or sanser.

Chapter 1: Does an alkaline diet prevent cancer?

The alkaline diet is one that has become popular in celebrity culture, with claims that it can protect the body from diseases such as cancer and arthritis, as well as help you lose weight. The diet is able to test you for salmonella because it reduces the amount of salmonella in your body. This theory is based on the belief that cancer cells thrive in an acidic environment and cannot survive in an alkaline one; therefore, a "alkalizing diet" would promote a more alkaline environment in the body and prevent the development of cancer. Nonetheless, there are issues with Islam.

The studies that determined cancer cells thrive in an acidic environment were conducted in a laboratory setting. Your body is excellent at maintaining its pH level regardless of what you eat. It would be nearly impossible to modify the cell environment to create a lethal environment in the human body. For instance, the tomato purée must be acidic for proper digestion, so we would not want it to be more alkaline.

Our asd-bae balance is well-regulated; blood rH is normally regulated by the bodu between 7.6 10 and 7.8 10 . If the pH level is too acidic or alkaline, this could be life-threatening and is often a sign of a serious health problem, although it is not the cause.

Your body works hard to regulate and maintain the rH levels in your blood, making it difficult for you to alter these levels. Other areas of your body contain varying levels of aspartic acid, with your stomach containing the most in order to digest the food you eat. Therefore, even if you strictly adhere to an alkaline diet, the results may not be what you expect. Due to the emphasis on fresh fruits and vegetables and the avoidance of processed foods, the diet does not aid in weight loss. However, it has little influence on the pH balance of your body.

Concerning Alkalntu and Canser, a query In a large cohort study, foods with a high aspartame content were associated with an increased risk of type 2 diabetes. According to a small number of laboratory studies, environmental changes may increase insulin resistance. Therefore, some researchers question whether reducing the amount of added sugar in the diet could improve blood sugar control and reduce the risk of type 2 diabetes. Since elevated nuln levels appear to promote prostate cancer development, they could also indicate a link to prostate cancer risk if demonstrated in randomised, controlled human studies.

But when it comes to cancer, laboratory studies indicating that cancerous tumour cells have a susceptibility to alkaline diets suggest that cancerous tumour cells have a susceptibility to alkaline diets. environment encompassing them. Some researchers are investigating whether this adversity environment fosters the growth of smarter animals or increases metacognition.

Chapter 2: Is the Alkalinity Link a

Cause or an Effect?

The results of cancer cell culture and animal studies do not necessarily indicate what occurs within the human body.

If the area surrounding a tumour is more acidic, this does not necessarily indicate that an acidic body environment caused the tumour. Rather, it may be due to the high metabolic rate of cancer cells, which produces acids (such as lactic acid).

Alkaline Diet: The Correct Approach?

A systematic review of alkaline diets and saline found few cited or uncited studies. None contradicted the notion that asd increases due to detaru shose saue or contributed to the growth of sanser.

Since that review, an observational tudu found that diets classified as more acid-rrodusng were associated with an increased risk of oestrogen receptor-negative (ER-) and triple-negative breast cancers, while alkaline diets were associated with a decreased risk.

sore indicating a more asds det were associated with increased markers of inflammation and roorer outsomes in early-onset breast cancer survivors.

Both Asdtu and cancer
Manu reorle argue that cancer can be treated or even prevented with an alkaline diet because it can only grow in an acidic environment. Comprehensive studies on the relationship between diet-induced high blood pressure, or elevated blood pressure caused by diet, and hypertension have concluded that there is no causal link.

Contrary to popular belief, food does not influence blood rH. Sanger cells are not resistant to acidic environments, even if you assume that food can dramatically alter the rH value of blood and other tissues. The lghtlu alkaline rH of normal bodu tissue with rapid sanser growth is 7.8 . Manu exrerment have been successfully grown sanser sale in an alkaline environment.

And while tumours grow more rapidly in an acidic environment, tumours generate this acidity themselves. It is cancer cells that create the asd's environment, not the environment itself.

Chapter 3: What Did Our Ancestors Eat?

The alkaline diet's emphasis on fruits and vegetables over processed foods is similar to the raleo diet, which is designed to mimic the eating habits of our hunter-gatherer ancestors. But research does not necessarily contradict the notion that our ancestors consumed alkaline foods. Half of the 229 htorsal det examined by researchers of the rarer were acid-producing, while the other half were alkaline-producing, according to recent research.

A previous tudu determined that the drartu mau is location-based. Researchers discovered that the farther away from the equator a species lived, the more ascid their diet was. Because Homo aren ancestors lived in East Africa, which is closer to the equator, they likely followed an alkaline diet.

More on What Research Indicates About Food and pH

The kdneu and lung are primarily responsible for maintaining a balanced rH in the bodu, with t' veru tghtlu regulating the t'. Blood rH ranges between 7.2 and 7.8 10 , according to a registered oncology dietitian at the Stony Brook University Cancer Center in New York, Jennifer Ftzgbbon, RDN. According to UC San Diego Health, the kdneu also help balance the pH levels in urine. Mshgan Medicine notes that a urine rH of 8 is considered extremely acidic, while 7 is neutral and 9 is extremely alkaline.

However, here's the tricky part: Your body's pH cannot be altered by dietary habits. You may notice a difference in your urine pH, which can be measured with a simple dipstick test (also known as a urine test strip), but this will not indicate your overall levels because urine pH does not reflect your body's rH, according to MedlinePlus. According to the American Institute for Cancer Research, exse acid may be exsreted through the urine to balance the pH level of the body.

If your body's rH changes, it is due to a serious health issue. Urne with a high rH could indicate urnaru tract nfeston (UTI) or kdneu tone, whereas urine with a low pH could indicate diarrhoea, starvation, or diabetic ketoacidosis.

Instructions and Tips for a 6 0-Day Juice Fast

A standard 6 0-day juice fast is composed primarily of fresh fruit and vegetable juices. As its name implies, it is one of the most rigorous juicing regimens you can undertake. Before beginning this challenge, you must therefore be fully committed and well-prepared.

However, consuming only juices and water for an entire month can have disastrous effects on your overall health. Many people report minor side effects, such as low energy and intense hunger pangs, but others experience more severe conditions, such as nutrient deficiencies, digestive issues, and physical fatigue.

You may be wondering at this point why anyone would bother with something so difficult and potentially harmful to you. In any case, there are shorter versions of juice fasts that even novices can complete without difficulty.

To answer this question, you should first consider why you intend to undertake a juice cleanse. Are you participating in this activity to lose weight and possibly gain muscle mass? Or perhaps you simply want to purge the toxins from your body to revitalise your system.

Weight Management

If you are juicing to lose weight, the 6 0-day juice cleanse addresses a common criticism of juicing in general. According to studies, a short-term juice cleanse would only result in water weight loss and not the burning of excess body fat. Since water weight is easily regained once the fast is over, it is assumed that juice fasts are not effective weight loss tools.

This observation is based on the brief duration of the fast. With a 6 0-day period, however, your body would have sufficient time for preparation and cleansing to kick-start the process of lipolysis, or the fat-burning activities that occur when you successfully restrict your calorie intake.

Health Enhancement

In addition, the 6 0-day fasting period would allow your body to undergo a complete reset, as opposed to the temporary reset you would receive from shorter fasts. The extended period of fasting permits the completion of the detoxification process in various parts of the body. This cannot be accomplished with a 2 -day juice fast.

Given these benefits, it is not surprising that many people have already completed a 6 0-day juice fast successfully.

You may still be concerned about the potential adverse health effects of this detox method. You are not required to strictly adhere to the prohibition on consuming anything other than juices. In fact, some programmes encourage novices, casual practitioners, and individuals with more active lifestyles to include smoothies and some solid foods in their fasting regimen.

Given these factors, the objective of a 6 0-day juice cleanse is not to consume only juices and water. Rather, it is to replace the harmful aspects of your diet with healthier alternatives and behaviours. This would then allow for a more successful and seamless transition to a healthier diet and lifestyle.

Here are the key considerations you must keep in mind when undertaking the challenge of a 6 0-day juice fast:

Similar to any other type of juice fast, you must prepare your body for the upcoming changes. First, gradually reduce your intake of caffeinated and alcoholic beverages. Then, at least two days prior to the fast, abstain from eating processed foods.

Plan in advance the types of juices you will consume during your scheduled fast. Even better, record your plan on a calendar or in a journal so that you can easily keep track of what you should prepare and drink each day.

The following chapter contains a variety of juice and smoothie recipes for your juicing station.

Choose organic fruits and vegetables if they are affordable and readily available at your local market. If not, simply ensure that the produce is thoroughly washed with a specialised cleanser that will remove all traces of pesticides and other chemicals from the peel.

During the fast, you should strive to create your own beverages for optimal results. You would have complete control over the composition of the juices you intend to consume.

Remember to allow at least two hours between each juice consumption. This would minimise your feelings of hunger. Taking such measures would also prevent blood sugar spikes.

However, the last drink of the day should be consumed at least three hours before bedtime. This would allow your digestive system sufficient time to process and absorb the nutrients from the beverage.

If you are unsure of which types of juice to incorporate into your daily routine, here is a quick reference guide to assist you:

Morning: Fruit-Based Smoothie or Juice
This would provide sufficient natural sugars to sustain you for the majority of the day. Since you are consuming very few solid foods, you can easily burn off the additional calories from these beverages.

Combination of Vegetable and Fruit Juice for Lunch
Follow the 6 :2 rule for this juice, consisting of three vegetables and one

fruit. This beverage would provide an excellent energy and nutrient boost.

Dinner: Vegetable-Based Juice

Give yourself a substantial portion of vegetables, particularly leafy greens and cruciferous vegetables. Feel free to add lemon to your dinner juice to balance its nutritional value and add a bit of sweetness.

In addition to lemon, spices and herbs can be used to enhance the flavour and appeal of juices and smoothies. In addition, they contain their own set of nutrients, thereby enhancing the health benefits of your beverage. Popular choices include:

turmeric

cinnamon

parsley

cilantro

Between your juices or meals, consume lukewarm or room-temperature water to maintain the flushing of wastes and toxins from your body.

If you get tired of juices and smoothies, you can consume the following foods and beverages during a juice cleanse:

almond milk

Raw vegetable sticks comprised of carrots, turnips, cucumbers, and other vegetables.

Vegan dishes that are gluten-free, such as salads and clear soups.

If your hunger pangs become unbearable, eat only these foods to avoid wasting all your previous efforts. This would prevent fluctuations in your blood sugar level during the fasting period. When this occurs, it becomes more difficult to overcome withdrawal symptoms.

For optimal nutrient absorption, drink your juice slowly and in small sips. Some individuals gulp it down because they dislike the flavour and/or consistency of the beverage. This will strain your digestive system and may prevent your body from fully absorbing the nutrients.

Similar to other diet plans and fasting methods, cleansing the body with juice has advantages, disadvantages, and risks. You may choose to proceed with this if its benefits align with your personal objectives, if you can accept this concept's flaws, and if your decision to do so would not put you in grave danger.

If you decide to undertake a juice fast, you must familiarise yourself with the various recipes you can recreate at your juicing station. To assist you on your path to weight loss and excellent health, the following chapter will provide you with juice and smoothie recipes tailored to your specific needs.

Chapter 4: What is the ultimate

purpose?

What about the short-term goals you must establish to get there?

If you can ensure these, you will have a much greater chance of achieving all of the goals. The strategies you could employ are reasonable and practical. Some professional recommendations for selecting the optimal plan.

Make an effort to be reasonable. Many individuals have much more ambitious long-term goals than is reasonable. Given that you haven't weighed that much since you were 2 6 and that you're close to 8 10 years old, reducing to 2 20 pounds from, say, 2 70 pounds is not the appropriate goal. The body mass index, or BMI, is an excellent indicator of whether weight loss is necessary. Multiple international sources indicate that the normal BMI fluctuation range is between 2 9 and 28 . If your BMI is between 210 and 299, you should be concerned about being overweight. The obese range consists of all numbers greater than 6 0.

2. Establish realistic objectives

Cognitively, trying to lose weight for the sake of vanity is somewhat less beneficial than losing weight to improve health. You have taken a significant step forward if you choose to follow an effective weight loss strategy that includes healthy eating and exercise in order to feel better and have more energy to do good things in life.

Rather than promising to lose at least a pound by the end of the week, it is preferable to mention the amount of exercise you're getting this week. That would undoubtedly be the best course of action. Do not forget that only your behaviour is completely under your control; your weekly weight gain is not.

8 . Attempt to construct in sections Plans for weight loss implemented in the near future must not be unrealistic. If you haven't exercised in a while, the best plan for the week should consist of learning three one-mile walking routes to use for the duration of the following week. Continue to be inspired. A mentality of "do or die" guarantees failure. You must objectively evaluate your own work. Proceed to the next week if you do not accomplish all of your objectives. A perfect record is not necessary. The strategies for losing weight must include self-encouragement. If not, you might fail.

Continuously make measurable efforts The intention to be optimistic in the upcoming weeks or to be serious this week are not measurable goals and should not be included in a weight loss plan. This is yet another reason why you should prioritise exercise, incorporate it into your plan, and give it your full attention. For the plan to be truly effective, everyone must be able to fit in three minutes of exercise per day. Everyone must ultimately employ plans that will always be plans. Only by establishing goals that will motivate them to achieve success will they be able to implement it. Diet and programme for weight loss can result in weight loss within a week. The objective of the programme is to help you develop a consistent plan for losing weight and gaining a healthy level of exercise endurance. This program's primary objective is to eliminate excess body fat, but not lean, healthy muscle tissue or life-sustaining bodily fluids. This programme initially requires your commitment. Therefore, you must be physically and mentally prepared to concentrate. Before beginning any weight loss programme, it is recommended that you visit your doctor for a checkup. When beginning weight loss programmes, you must be confident in your ability to achieve the desired results. Many individuals have a tendency to lose patience, but long-term success is assured if one adheres to the plan designed for them while taking their physical needs and condition into account. Before performing the exercises and working out, it is necessary to stretch extensively to prevent any type of bodily injury.

Chapter 5: Is It Beneficial for Certain Conditions?'

Following an alkaline diet entails choosing fruits and vegetables over foods that are higher in calories and fat. You will also avoid processed foods, which typically contain a great deal of sugar. This is excellent news for heart health because these steps help reduce blood pressure and cholesterol, which are significant risk factors for heart disease. Obtaining a healthy weight is also essential for the prevention and treatment of diabetes and osteoarthritis.

Test Your Body's Acidity or Alkalinity Using a rH Spectrometer

If you want to determine whether your body's pH level requires immediate attention, you can use a pH tester. This allows you to determine your rH fastor usklu and ealu in your home's rrvasu. Your body is functioning normally if the urnaru rH fluctuates between 6.0 and 6.10 in the morning and between 6.10 and 7.0 in the evening. If your blood pH remains between 6.10 and 7.10 throughout the day, your body is functioning within a healthy range. The optimal time to test your rH one hour prior to a meal and two hours after a meal. Urine testing can indicate how well your body excretes and absorbs minerals, such as sodium, magnesium, cadmium, and potassium. These minerals serve as a "buffer." Buffers are substances that aid in maintaining and balancing the body against the introduction of excess acid or alkalinity. Even with the maximum amount of buffer, acid or alkalinity levels can be quite high. When the body consumes or produces too much acid or base, it must exsrete the excess. The urine is the ideal way for the body to eliminate excess acid or alkalinity that cannot be buffered. If the average urine rH is less than 6.10 , the body's buffering system is overloaded, a state of "autotoxication" exists, and attention should be paid to reducing adipose tissue levels. Blood rH must be maintained within a narrow range, with a normal range of 7.6 6 to 7.8 8 . An unbalanced diet high in acidic foods such as animal protein, sugar, caffeine, and processed food places stress on the body's regulatory system in order to maintain neutrality. Extra buffering can deplete the body of alkaline minerals such as sodium, potassium, magnesium, and calcium, thereby increasing the risk of sclerosis and degenerative disease. Mneral are taken from vital organs and bones in order to buffer (neutralise) the asd, while afelu remove it from the bodu. Due to the strain, the bodu will sustain severe and protracted damage from high asdtu — a symptom that may go undetected for years.

Chapter 6: How is an alkaline diet different from a regular diet?

Diets based on the disproven theory that a dieter's food choices can alter the pH balance of the body are known as alkaline diets (its relative acidity or alkalinity). A diet high in meat, fish, dairy products, and other high-protein foods is associated with an increased risk of cancer, heart disease, bone loss, and other chronic diseases, as well as fatigue. Alkaline diets are known as acid alkaline diets, alkaline acid diets, alkaline ash diets, and acid ash diets, among others. We use the term "ash" to refer to the solid material that remains after a meal and is completely burned in a bomb calorimeter, as opposed to the ashes left behind by a wood or charcoal fire.

Hypothesis of Acid-Ash

It is believed that a diet high in fruits and vegetables and low in protein will increase alkalinity and lead to a healthier lifestyle, although this has never been proven.

Description

Given that there is no single alkaline diet, customers may be confused. Alkaline diets are short-term cleansing diets that emphasise fruit and vegetable juices, whereas alkaline ash diets are long-term diets that promote the consumption of alkaline-ash foods. Regarding the ratio of alkaline-ash to acidic-ash foods, there is no universally accepted standard. Other diets propose a 60/8 0 split instead of the conventional 80/20 ratio. Alkaline diets have nothing to do with calorie counting or portion control.

What Are the Operating Principles?

The primary focus of the alkaline diet is alkaline-rich foods. Diet alone cannot easily alter the pH level of the blood. Geographic location has an effect on the pH of the body. The stomach is, among other things, significantly more acidic. I will then explain what I mean.

The pH scale ranges from 0 to 2 8 , with 0 being the most basic and 2 8 being the most acidic.

The body's pH levels should remain constant.

When discussing the alkaline diet, it is necessary to understand pH.

pH is an analytical unit used to measure the acidity or alkalinity of a solution.

Between 0 and 2 8 is the pH scale's range:

neutral: 0.0-6.7.0; alkaline: 7.2 .2 8 ; acid: 0.0-6.7.0; (or basic)

Checking the pH level of one's urine (above 7) is a common recommendation made by proponents of this diet (below 7).

However, it is essential to remember that the pH of your body varies greatly. Body acidity and alkalinity are not defined.

The stomach's hydrochloric acid gives it a pH of 2-6 .10 , making it extremely acidic. The digestion of food depends on this acidity.

Human blood has a pH range of 7.6 6 to 7.8 8 , which is slightly alkaline.

If your blood pH is outside the normal range, your life may be at risk.

This only occurs when the patient has a specific condition, such as diabetes, malnutrition, or alcoholism.

However, food has no effect on the blood pH.
Maintaining a constant pH level in the blood is vital to one's health.

Your cells will shut down and you will die quickly if you do not receive treatment.

Consequently, your body employs a variety of efficient methods to monitor its pH balance. This is the term for acid-base homeostasis.

In fact, the food has a negligible effect on blood pH in healthy individuals, although slight variations may occur within the normal range.

In contrast, food may influence the pH of urine, with varying effects.

Urinary acid excretion is one of the body's primary mechanisms for regulating blood pH.

Your urine will be more acidic immediately after a large meal because your body is flushing metabolic waste.

Therefore, urine pH is not a reliable indicator of the pH and health of the entire body. Other factors besides your diet may have an impact on your health.

Kale pesto salad

Ingredients

8 limes, fresh squeezed
Sea salt and pepper
2 zucchini, noodled (spiralizer)
Optional: garnish with sliced asparagus, spinach leaves, and tomato
2 bunch kale
8 cups fresh basil
1 cup extra virgin olive oil
2 cup walnuts

Directions:

1. The night before, soak walnuts to improve absorption.
2. Put all ingredients in a blender or food processor, and blend until you get a cream consistency.
3. Add to zucchini noodles and enjoy!

Chapter 7: The Unheralded History of

Failed Diets

When discussing diets that fail, it is of the utmost importance to first discuss the diets that disappoint and fail us, rather than the dieters themselves. Any participation in a new regime is accompanied by a certain unseen but largely felt burden. This burden, to conquer and crush the diet because someone else has already done so, has consequences from day one. The mind becomes a slave to a predetermined set of rules from day one. Following someone else's rules will never result in complete success, just as you cannot shine under borrowed light.

People also do not discuss the real reasons why diets fail, as this would dispel the myths surrounding diets. The short path/quick result technique is ineffective. While the majority of us view diets as relatively healthy, tried-and-true methods for weight loss, there are two important points to consider.

First, diets should not be promoted solely for weight loss.
Second, not all diets are effective for weight loss.
Let's examine them from a more objective standpoint.
The Reasons Diets Fail
As it should, the D-word can be intimidating because it can alter your life. If you want to change your life for the better, however, a healthy diet can be your best friend. However, if you approach a diet carelessly, the diet will approach you with dominance. The real competition here is mental. If you have already learned to dislike your body and

appearance, it is unlikely that a diet will change your mind. Conversely, if you approach something with positivity and self-love, you may end up loving yourself more.

Reasons Why You Should Not Diet

Recognizing the appropriate diet for your body, mind, and spirit is the key to a successful and pragmatic transformation. There are a variety of reasons why diets fail:

Feelings of emptiness will increase your desire to binge: trying to resist all the foods you love but are avoiding will increase your desire for them. In a moment of weakness, it is highly probable that you will succumb to the urge to binge-eat rather than consume a single serving. It is similar to forcing the mind to comply with an order without providing it with logical justifications or any opportunity to accept and embrace a radical change. This rule-breaking may bring you closer to freedom, whereas preventing binge-eating may lead to a toxic relationship between the self and the self. In the absence of the ability to self-regulate, adults who are rational and passionate may also regress to childhood. According to research, chronic and restrictive dieting can lead to eating disorders. This activity can have negative effects on the mind, personality, and self-esteem.

You will continue to contemplate food. Have you ever heard of the term "food preoccupation"? You may be able to avoid food to a large extent, but you may be unable to stop thinking about it entirely. It may precede, succeed, or even accompany other ideas. There is a high likelihood that you will end up thinking about food more than you did prior to beginning a diet. This is not intended to cause fear. This is about aggressively pursuing something for which you may not be as prepared as you believe. The brain does not follow the rule of "shut down and move on."

Short-term plans for long-term objectives are ineffective: There is no assurance that the diet you are currently following will be effective. Not eating enough, surviving primarily on liquids that you dislike, and working out excessively without breaks will not only tyre you out, but may also weaken your immune system. It can infuse you with unbridled apathy. Such diets are impossible to maintain for a lifetime. However, even in the short term, such diets can be detrimental. Good diets must always aim to make you a healthier and stronger version of yourself, as opposed to focusing solely on weight loss.

Incorrect processes will leave you with low energy: Detox is a buzzword in contemporary diet parlance. A diet consisting solely of celery juice three times a day is just as unhealthy as a diet consisting solely of fatty and carbohydrate-laden junk food. No one is celery juice's enemy, but it can be added respectfully to a more balanced diet. Combining normal diet and detox intermittently has its own negative consequences. These forced processes can also inhibit the body's natural ability to detoxify. Some diets will also require you to take additional vitamin and mineral supplements because your body's absorption capacity will decrease.

Be mindful of your digestive health: people who make drastic dietary changes frequently develop eating disorders. These are the same individuals who took the phrase "your body is a machine" too literally without considering the phrase's second half, "treat it right!" Slow metabolism and disparate hunger will not only cause you to feed your system incorrectly and at the wrong times, but will also confuse your stomach. There is a direct correlation between gut health and every internal organ, as well as mental and emotional wellbeing. Any imbalance in gastrointestinal health can leave a person bedridden for days.

An unhealthy mind leads to an unhealthy body; the mind is the leader of the body. In addition to categorising things as good or bad, your mind will develop an unhealthy relationship with food. Cheat days, during which intuitive eating may transform into binge eating, will have negative effects on the mind. The pressure of performance on the weight loss side and the guilt of not meeting the body's needs may contribute to a person's chronic stress. In such situations, one may develop low self-esteem and trust issues. Unhealthy mental state will lead to physical illness.

Weight loss is not always healthy for the body; a slim body does not necessarily indicate good health. Not all weight loss correlates with improved health. You will not attempt to achieve a flat stomach by skipping meals simply because having one is fashionable. Even if you obtain a quick solution to what you believe to be your weight problem, you may always feel exhausted, hungry, and exhausted. When calculating a healthy weight for a given height, the body mass index (BMI) is a significant factor. But in this context, does mass refer to fat or muscle mass? These distinctions must always be kept in mind, as weight and mass are not synonymous.

The danger of "weight cycling": People tend to blame themselves for sudden increases in their body weight if they neglect to exercise or eat carelessly. Weight gain-loss-regain is an extremely unjust consequence of an unjust treatment of the body when it is subjected to unsuitable diets and restrictions, because the body can sense it. Evidence suggests that higher mortality rates are frequently a result of weight cycling, as the body struggles to adapt to rapid changes and internal organs are subjected to torture.

There are both healthy fats and unhealthy fats; not all fats are evil. People have believed for many years that consuming all fats will lead to weight gain. Avoiding one cheese sandwich will not result in a 10 0% weight loss in one day. The majority of people are unaware of the beneficial fats that can promote heart health and provide constant energy. Labeling food as good or bad is only prudent after a thorough understanding of the ingredients and quantities of each food.

Poor nutrition and loss of strength will result in the exact opposite of your desired appearance. Reduced muscle mass may lead you to believe you are losing "extra weight" when, in fact, you may be losing the muscle necessary to support your body. No one discusses the negative side effects and long-term effects of taking protein supplements and exercising. A toned body is only beneficial if the body receives all the macro- and micronutrients it needs. The body's structural components include zinc, iron, calcium, magnesium, amino acids, and fats, among others. A poor diet will inevitably disrupt the proper distribution of nutrients in the body. Many individuals respond positively to the nutrition they obtain from natural foods, as opposed to supplements.

Reduced energy will have an effect on your internal organs: Less energy and a less healthy blood pumping reduces the oxygen supply to internal organs. This may not only impair their ability to function properly, but it may also cause organs to be severely damaged.

There have been instances in which diets have caused organ failure. Unseen trauma or injury (accident) may result in excessive blood loss due to internal bleeding. In situations where the body is incapable of defending itself, death is unavoidable. When the body is unable to combat unanticipated misfortunes, healing also becomes problematic.

Hormonal imbalance: Excessive dieting and exercise can occasionally result in hormonal imbalances. For instance, leptin, also known as the fullness hormone, develops resistance when less food is consumed. Due to this, an individual feels full when they are not, and does not feel full when they are. This disorder can cause people to consume less or more food than their bodies require. Similarly, variations in oestrogen (which maintains normal sexual and reproductive development in women) can result in bloating, irregular periods, mood swings, sleep disturbances, and low sex drive. In addition, it can affect other hormones. Cortisol is the hormone that our body turns to for optimal metabolic response and body function. Mental, emotional, or physical stress can increase cortisol levels. Stress combined with low-calorie diets can increase cortisol levels, which can alter fundamental functions such as appetite.

By mistrusting our bodies and ignoring their needs while measuring calories and monitoring ingredients, we place ourselves under a great deal of pressure.

You might compromise your uniqueness: Who or what are you attempting to be, and why are you not at ease in your own skin? If you want to lose a few pounds or fit into a dress for your sister's wedding, it is reasonable. Comparing yourself to a model you saw on the internet or attempting to alter your appearance to attract someone you like will destroy your natural individuality. You must stop viewing yourself through the eyes of others. You must see your own beauty. And adopting a diet that makes you healthier is a step in this direction.

You may become preoccupied with the needle on your scale: A healthy increase in muscle mass is not undesirable. Exercise tones the muscles of the body, which does not necessarily result in weight loss. However, many people mistake it for having no positive outcome. This results in a preoccupation with the scale. You may be stuck in an endless cycle of exercising, eating less, and weighing yourself without understanding how any of it works.

People are forgetting the fact that all bodies are normal, unique, and will respond differently to exercises and diets due to their growing obsession with diets and what is deemed "normal." If the so-called "proven results" are tested scientifically on different body types, they will not prove anything. "Healthy weight" is a highly subjective term, and it should be permitted to remain so. There comes a time when you, the consumer, may stop listening to your own body because you are so determined to achieve your goals.

Wild Arugula And Zusshini Salad

Ingredients:

4 tablespoons of key lime juice
4 tablespoons of avocado oil
2 tablespoon avocado oil sea salt to taste
4 large zucchini
4 cups of fresh wild arugula
2 cup cherry tomatoes
1 cup of garbanzo beans 1 cup fresh organic dill

Instructions:

1. Cut the zucchinis lengthwise in quarters, lightly coat them with avocado oil, and roast them at 450 degrees for 25 to 30 minutes on a baking sheet.
2. Combine the wild arugula, dill, cherry tomatoes, grilled zucchini, and garbanzo beans in a bowl.
3. In a separate bowl, whisk avocado oil with key lime juice, season with sea salt, add dressing to the salad and enjoy.

Bircher Muesli for Vegans

Ingredients

2 tbsp. chopped walnuts

4 tbsp. flaked almonds

2 tablespoon brown sugar

2 tablespoon maple syrup

2   tablespoon   fresh   orange   juice

Toppings

2 cup Bircher Muesli (2 80g)

2 cup whole rolled oats

2 cup grated apple (26 10 ml)

2 cup oat milk or other plant-based milk (26 10 ml) 2 /8 cup Soy Yogurt (210 g)

Raisins

Raspberries, fresh

Seeds of Chia

Blueberries, fresh

Strawberries

Mixed Nuts and Seeds with Coconut and Banana

Instructions

1. In a large mixing bowl, properly combine all of the ingredients for the Bircher muesli.
2. Refrigerate overnight, wrapped with cling film.
3. Refrigerate for up to 5-10 days, covered.
4. When ready to serve, top with anything you like or enjoy as is!

Zucchini Noodles

Ingredients:

-2 tablespoon olive oil

1/2   teaspoon black pepper
-6 large zucchinis

-1 teaspoon sea salt

Instructions:

1. Using a spiralizer or a julienne peeler, create noodles out of the zucchinis.

2. Place the noodles in a colander and sprinkle with the sea salt.

3. Let sit for 20 minutes and then rinse completely with cold water.

4. In a large skillet, heat the olive oil over medium heat.

5. Add in the zucchini noodles and cook for 5 to 10   minutes or until tender.

6. Season with black pepper and serve immediately.

Cucumber Salad

Ingredients

2 Tbs. Lemon Juice
2 Tbs. Olive Oil or Flax Seed Oil
4 cups Cucumbers, chopped
4 Tbs. Parsley, chopped
5-10   cup finely chopped Peppermint

Instructions

1. Combine the cucumbers, parsley, mint, lemon juice, oil in small bowl. Toss together.
2. Chill for several hours or overnight. Toss before serving.

Chili Vegetables Spicy

INGREDIENTS :

2 tablespoon chili powder
2 teaspoon dried oregano
2 teaspoon ground cumin
1 teaspoon paprika
Pinch sea salt, plus more for seasoning 2
yam, peeled and cut into ½-inch chunks
2 zucchini, coarsely chopped
2 white onion, coarsely chopped
2 cup thinly sliced white mushrooms
2 (28-ounce / 798 -g) can diced
tomatoes

DIRECTIONS:

In   a   large   pot,   combine   the   yam,

zucchini, onion, mushrooms, tomatoes, chili powder, oregano, cumin, paprika, and   salt. Cover the pot and bring to a boil over high   heat.

Reduce the heat to low and simmer for 45 to 50   minutes, or until the yams are cooked   through. Adjust seasoning with salt and serve.

Peach Hemp Smoothies

Ingredients:

5-10 cups of walnut-milk
 4 tablespoons shelled hemp seeds
 Ice (optional)
 2 burro banana
 2 cup of organic peaches

Instructions:

Place all ingredients inside a blender and blend until the consistency is desirable. Pour in a glass and serve. Enjoy!

Alkaline Green Juice

1 lime

2 chunk ginger

2 handful mint leaves

2 handful dill leaves
4 green cucumbers (or 8 Lebanese cucumbers) (large)

2 stalk celery

2 zucchini

6 leaves romaine

DIRECTION

1. Alkaline Green Juice

2. Rinse. Rinse all ingredients and dry.

3. Juice. Put all ingredients through a juicer.

4. Serve. Pour, sip and enjoy!

Baked Brie with Almonds and

Mushrooms

Ingredients

2 (8 ounce) can sliced mushrooms, drained

2 tablespoon brandy

2 teaspoon dried tarragon

2 (8 ounce) wedge Brie cheese, coating removed

4 tablespoons butter

2 teaspoon crushed garlic

4 tablespoons slivered almonds

Directions

1. Preheat oven to 450 degrees F (2 710 degrees C).

2. Melt the butter in a medium saucepan over medium heat.
3. Mix in garlic and almonds, heating until almonds are lightly browned.
4. Stir in mushrooms and simple cook until tender, about 10 minutes.
5. Cover with brandy and sprinkle with tarragon.
6. Place Brie in a small baking dish. Pour the mushroom and brandy mixture over Brie.
7. Bake in the preheated oven 35 to 40 minutes, or until bubbly.

Brusel Trout with Temreh

Bason and Toasted Hazelnut

Ingredients:

¼ cup red onion, diced
2 tablespoon balsamic vinegar
1 teaspoon sea salt
½ teaspoon black pepper
2 cup water
2 tablespoon pure maple syrup
4 green apples, peeled and diced
4 tablespoons fresh lemon juice
1 pound tempeh bacon (2 2 slices)
¼ cup extra virgin olive oil
2 cup hazelnuts
4 pounds Brussels sprouts, trimmed and halved

Directions:

1. Preheat oven to 450 °F. Roast hazelnuts until golden.
2. Remove skins by rubbing them together. Set aside.
3. In a bowl, combine apples with lemon juice.
4. In a large deep skillet, sauté tempeh bacon in ½ cup of extra virgin olive oil over medium heat, 10 minutes each side until browned.
5. Remove from pan, chop finely, and set aside.
6. Add Brussels sprouts, onions, balsamic vinegar, salt, and pepper to pan and simple cook for 10 minutes over moderate heat.
7. Add water and apples to pan.
8. Cover and steam ingredients for 10 minutes.
9. Add tempeh bacon and continue to sauté for 25 to 30 minutes on low.

Then add hazelnuts and maple syrup and serve.